D1450737

8 LESSONS LUPUS TAUGHT ME

FROM SURVIVING TO THRIVING WITH AUTOIMMUNE DISEASES

CallyRae Stone

BALBOA.
PRESS

A DIVISION OF HAY HOUSE

Balboa Press books may be ordered through booksellers or by contacting:

Balboa Press
A Division of Hay House
1663 Liberty Drive
Bloomington, IN 47403
www.balboapress.com
1 (877) 407-4847

Print information available on the last page.

ISBN: 978-1-5043-9740-7 (sc)
ISBN: 978-1-5043-9741-4 (e)

Balboa Press rev. date: 02/09/2018

To my husband Joff and my kids Jessica, Christopher, and Jenna;

Thank you for being my inspiration to be better and do better each day. You are the wind beneath my wings.

Contents

Acknowledgments

A special thank you to Debbie Gibbons and Brandi McMahon for editing and providing feedback for the attention to detail that I lack.

As these lessons are a compilation of my life experiences through my autoimmune journey, there is no way to reference, credit or acknowledge everyone who has been a part of this journey or made a contribution to this book. My only hope is that I can pay it forward and leave the road better than I found it.

My greatest acknowledgment is to my Father in Heaven and my Savior Jesus Christ who have made this journey possible and the lessons a series of blessings.

Finally, to acknowledge my family who have lived the journey with me and loved me both as a munching caterpillar and a soaring butterfly.

Introduction: My Story

My name is Cally Stone and at the time of completing this book I am 48 years old. My story of course begins at birth. However the relevant points of this experience, my autoimmune journey, begin at age 25 just as I completed my Masters of Science Degree in Speech Language Pathology.

Shortly after graduation, in what is called the Clinical Fellow Year, I experienced my first symptoms of rheumatoid arthritis (RA). I was diagnosed the following year after moving back to Boise in 1998. My thought was "I am too young to have arthritis" but rheumatoid arthritis ran in my family with both my mother and grandmother having RA so I didn't give it much more thought.

At that time in my scientific education I had learned about genetics and the fact that you were destined with the genetics from your DNA. In 1999, I began experiencing chronic infections that would not heal but morph from one thing into another. I would have bronchitis from October through May every year with a bronchial cough that would linger year-round. Sinus infections would morph into cellulitis and staph infections. Urinary tract infections would be complicated by yeast infections and vacillate back and forth as treatment for one would exacerbate the other.

Both my internist and gynecologist were perplexed and prescribing antibiotics, steroids, antifungals, and anti-inflammatories all of which would only give brief resolution until the "bug" would morph into another presentation. Finally, my internist determined that I had colonized staph in my sinuses from working in healthcare (by this time in hospitals and skilled nursing facilities for 5 years). When my sinuses would drain the staph was opportunistic and would take up residence wherever it would find an opportunity. It seemed like a plausible explanation and we all went with it for years as I would cycle through what seemed like an endless infection of one sort or another.

Finally in 2011, I had an outbreak of skin lesions. They weren't severe (especially in comparison to the gnarly infections I was used to). The lesions were relatively small and scattered randomly, or so I thought, on various places on my body. The largest one was on my scalp and was itchy but not painful. It was just an irritation on the crown of my head, so I couldn't really see the little bald spot. Other lesions were more painful so I had seen the doctor. She discounted it as another strange presentation with no explanation or solution. So I continued to ignore them and went about my life, irritated but not sick.

Then I had the most bizarre outbreak in my mouth. At first I didn't notice anything, but my mouth HURT like it was on fire with gasoline. It hurt to eat, it hurt to drink, it hurt to talk, and it hurt like nothing else! As I examined my mouth (I am a speech therapist after all. I know how to do an oral exam!) I noticed white horizontal lines in my gums and the inside of my cheeks. My gums were red and inflamed.

I had never seen anything like that in a patient's mouth. My daughter was in college as a dental assistant student so I had her take a peak. "Have you seen anything like that in your books?" "No" she said. So the two of us sat down and started researching on the internet these white lines and inflamed gums and came up with "Oral Lichen

Planus" as the perfect self-diagnoses by Cally & Jessica Stone! The only problem was, for treatment (and a "real" diagnosis) it said you should see your dentist. Absolutely NOT!

My mouth was so sore there was no way I was stepping foot in a dental office let alone a dental chair. I kept searching and found that a dermatologist could also diagnose and treat Oral Lichen Planus. That sounded much gentler to me so I made an appointment feeling quite confident that this was merely a technicality to get my hands on the prescription I needed to relieve the firestorm of pain in my mouth.

When I met with the dermatologist and gave her my health history and recent bout of irritating skin lesions but "the only reason I'm here is for you to diagnose this Oral Lichen Planus so I can get relief". She said the craziest thing I had heard in my entire life.

"I think you have Lupus"

"WHAT? No I don't have Lupus. I feel better than I have ever felt in my entire adult life! I have lost 70 pounds, I exercise regularly and have energy that I haven't had since I was 16 years old. I don't even have arthritis pain any more. I just have Oral Lichen Planus. It's the only thing wrong with me."

So she tricked me! She convinced me that it would be prudent to do a biopsy of the lesion on my scalp since it wasn't healing and had been there for about 6 months. As a redhead with freckles and siblings with skin cancer, I agreed that it probably was a good idea to make sure I didn't have skin cancer on the top of my head. So she popped a biopsy out and sent it off to the lab.

She gave me some lip service about the Oral Lichen Planus and a prescription for Miracle Mouthwash (a pharmacist compound that is used with AIDS patients who get similar painful mouth sores). Yikes! I came to the dermatologist physically feeling better than I had ever felt as an adult but with one heck of a sore mouth and left being told I had Lupus and was given a prescription for AIDS patients.

The dermatologist called me a week later and said,

> "Your biopsy results came back as unrecognizable so I am sending it off to another lab."

> "OK"

I wasn't really sure how I was supposed to respond or what I should have asked so that was all I could come up with. As I thought about it, I realized "well at least it's not cancer, because that would have been recognizable, right?"

The Miracle Mouthwash was helping a bit, because it basically numbed my mouth, but the lines and inflammation weren't calming down. I was just happy to have something that gave me some relief and on with life I went.

When I went in for my follow-up appointment with the dermatologist she shared with me that the lab results had come back from the second lab. They were positive for both Systemic Lupus Erythematosus and Oral Lichen Planus; both were autoimmune (AI) diseases. She then let me know that AI diseases often travel in packs, when you get one you will often have another. She laid out the treatment options of super antibiotic treatment, chemo therapy drugs, and steroids that may manage the symptoms of the Lupus and Lichen Planus.

> "Um, NO! I mean no thank you. I have patients and family members on these drugs and the side effects are awful. Remember, I said I FEEL better than I

have in my entire adult life. I am healing my body. This is not new; it is just a new diagnosis, and a new morph on an old problem."

I left the doctor's office with a standing order for Miracle Mouthwash, some topical steroids for the skin lesions, and a follow up appointment; but respectfully declined the aggressive allopathic medical approach I had become disenfranchised with because it hadn't helped "heal" my Arthritis or infections up to now, why would it now?

To understand my confident decline to the traditional standard approach to Lupus and Autoimmune Diseases, I'll take you back a few years to 2008. I'll share this part of my story in more detail in Lesson 2 but for the sake of continuity in this history you need to know that fruits and vegetables in a capsule changed my life and became a catalyst on this journey, before I even knew I was on the Autoimmune Highway. What I was experiencing as a miracle of healing my Rheumatoid Arthritis became much more than that as I continued to read everything I could get my hands on about nutritional healing and cellular health. I had learned that I was constantly growing ALL new cells in my body and I could either make healthy cells or sick cells based on the choices I made about how I fed those cells.

When I returned home from the doctor's office, I had confidence that I was already on the road to healing and that this was not new. As I researched Lupus and Lichen Planus I went through a number of feelings and reactions from fear to realization and even facing mortality. I realized that I DID in fact have the diseases she had diagnosed but when I looked back at what I now recognized as the cyclical nature of flare ups in autoimmune I could trace it all the way back to 1999. I had lived with Lupus symptoms undiagnosed for 12 years. Only the Lichen Planus was new to me. Then I realized that maybe the Rheumatoid Arthritis diagnosis was incorrect; maybe it was just the pain of Lupus, and I had it even longer.

Further study and living in my body with awareness now helped to me to recognize the difference between the Arthritis pain and the Lupus pain, they are distinct and different.

So fast forward to 2017 when I finally complete my story, or at least complete it for now. Maybe it's just a status update with the lessons that the autoimmune diseases have taught me (so far).

Lessons that I by no means expected to learn and hope to share with others to ease their suffering or possibly offer hope and guidance. Lessons that I wish I would have found on the internet when I was researching Lupus; because it was terrifying, and not at all hopeful, to receive these diagnoses and to see the pain and suffering and death in the literature and "support groups".

I have maintained my health and vitality since late 2008 with very few prescription medications, and then only for brief periods. I no longer have the chronic infections or debilitating flares that left me in bed recovering for weeks and even months. I have not been cured of Rheumatoid Arthritis, Systemic Lupus Erythematosus, or Oral Lichen Planus but I do manage them very effectively so that most people have no idea I have any disease let alone this lovely trio.

These are the 8 Lessons Lupus taught me. They are not the only lessons but they have been the most surprising and transformational for me. They are the lessons that have helped me reclaim my life and my destiny. You may notice some overlap within the lessons or some circling back. Unfortunately, I can be strong willed or slow to learn a lesson and so it will resurface in another way or at another time. Ultimately, the repetition gets through to me and clarity and change finally follow. I hope you enjoy the journey and find hope in healing and transformation.

LESSON 1

Your Genetics Are Not Your Destiny

As I was growing up, I had a healthy active family. I was the youngest of four children, trailing 15, 12 and 9 years behind my siblings. I don't have many childhood memories of my siblings. Most of the memories are just of them grown up as adults coming over to visit or work with my Dad on the farm. My parents farmed 30 acres in rural Idaho but Dad also worked as the concrete plant manager and travelled frequently. Mom was a stay-at-home mom that ruled with an iron fist, holding down the fort (I guess in this case farm) while my Dad was at work. They were both very hard working, proud, morally strong, independent people who expected the same of their children.

My mom and maternal grandmother both had Rheumatoid Arthritis so that was just normal. They were still very active and productive people. My maternal grandfather had died from a tree trimming accident on the ranch at age 72, clearly he was healthy and able-bodied climbing trees to the end. My mom had a congenital heart condition that was repaired prior to my birth. Mom had always had health issues but they weren't anything that kept her down. They were just her normal. I don't remember my Dad ever missing a day of work or even having a cold. Both of my paternal grandparents were diabetics; but I remember a cupboard full of pop always available when I would visit as well as a trip to the corner bait shop to get candy. Their diabetes clearly did not affect their lifestyle. My paternal grandfather also died at age 72 but after multiple heart attacks over many years.

As I got older, I chose to go to college for my Masters of Science Degree in Speech Language Pathology (SLP). I studied developmental milestones, anatomy and physiology, the disease processes for the speech sound systems, the oral motor system and the brain. As I studied I became very fascinated with the medical side of SLP and specialized in brain injury rehabilitation and neurological rehabilitation for conditions such as stroke, degenerative diseases and traumatic brain injury. I loved learning and had a lot of understanding of the brain anatomy and physiology as well as neuroplasticity.

In my professional climbing up the medical "corporate" ladder there were great recognition and accolades for being very busy, productive, working long hours, taking work home, volunteering for leadership and projects. Burning the candle at both ends and being a super-woman was rewarded. For me all that was normal. That is what I had watched my mother and father do. They were very hard working. That was how I was taught. Be the best. Do more. Be more. There is never enough. You do not take time for yourself. If you are hurting you just suck it up and drive on. That is normal. You have to keep functioning because you have to provide and the more you provide the better you are doing.

I was wired to believe that the more you do the more worthwhile you are. It's normal to hurt, it's normal to be tired, and it's normal to be sick. That's how everybody is.

As I was coming up to my 40th birthday, I had a realization. I was over 200 pounds on a 5'1" frame. I had chronic pain from rheumatoid arthritis which I had since I was 25. I would go to work, come home exhausted, order pizza for my family and go to bed. I realized that I needed to do something differently. This programming that I had would probably result in premature death or at best a poor quality of life.

I hadn't really thought about quality of life. I honestly didn't care if I lived or died. I was really tired of chronic pain and I had tried doctors and therapists and medications. Nothing had worked, so I just hadn't spent a lot of time thinking about it. I was just on autopilot. I was absolutely in survival mode.

As I came into this particular birthday, it was different. I saw my family, my siblings, who were in very poor health. My father had passed away at age 54, when I was 16, due to a "widow-maker", a massive deadly heart attack with no indication of heart disease or health concerns. He came home from working on a job site out of town and didn't feel well. Mom said she thought he needed to go the doctor. He said absolutely not so the next day on the way to another appointment my mom dropped him off at the ER. He was having a heart attack and had been all night. Three days later, the day he was scheduled to be discharged from the hospital, he had another attack and it took his life.

I was approaching the age of my oldest brother who passed away unexpectedly in his home at age 42, leaving behind a wife 7 months pregnant with their 8th child. His oldest son became the patriarch of the family; helping his mom as he finished high school, delaying a church mission until things stabilized, and the younger kids were older. His oldest daughter was also 16 when she lost her Dad; it still makes me cry to this day. The youngest three kids have few, if any, memories of their Dad. The coroner said it was complications of the flu but his family speculate of an undiagnosed heart condition or diabetes.

My other sister and brother were in and out of the hospital with serious conditions of asthma and diabetes. As my youngest brother reached his 40s, he was rushed to the hospital with what they thought was a heart attack but after further testing determined it was diabetic shock. His blood sugars were over 700 and the result was putting his body into a pseudo heart attack. That was when he learned he had diabetes. My sister struggled for years with allergies and had continual allergy shots for as long as I can remember. Now it was different. Now she had uncontrolled asthma that would land her in the emergency room not able to breathe. She was on long term prednisone and experimental shots to manage her asthma. Just to keep her breathing. They both looked like ticking time bombs to me, and I worried who was going to be next to leave their families prematurely.

Clearly, looking at health as a reason to slow down or take care of myself was not in my DNA. I thought I took care of myself. I don't smoke, I don't drink, and I don't do drugs. I am a great cook and I enjoy cooking for my family. However, my idea of health and what was normal at that time, I now know enough to have a completely different perspective on. I came into that birthday and thought "you know I need to make some changes…" I still remember my brother saying "fat, white and forty" that's why he had diabetes. Hmmm, I resembled that statement!

It was at that same time, as I came into that fateful birthday, that I was introduced to Juice Plus+. A whole foods plant based supplement full of anti-oxidants and phytonutrients which I wasn't getting. When I started getting this variety of 30 different fruits, vegetables and berries in my bloodstream my health changed and my eyes were opened. What I thought was normal, what I thought I needed to survive, and if I didn't survive it was ok, were all inaccurate. I had a 3 year old, a 13 year old and a 17 year old. I had to survive so that I could provide for them. That was my wiring. You survive, you get by.

Three years later, when I was 43, I was diagnosed with two more autoimmune diseases. I was diagnosed with Systemic Lupus Erythematosus and Oral Lichen Planus. What was crazy at that time was that I had lost 70 pounds; I had more energy than I'd ever had in my adult life and my chronic pain was gone. All because I was flooding my body with these antioxidants and it was hauling away the oxidative stress and free radical damage that had been stockpiling in my joints and attacking my skin and my organs. I was clearing this inflammation out. I felt so much better that I could not believe the Lupus diagnosis.

When I looked and researched a bit more, I realized that when I was diagnosed with Rheumatoid Arthritis in my 20s I didn't really believe that either. I thought I was too young. I realized it was in my family history so of course it's normal. Of course I'm going to have arthritis, it's in my genetics. But now we know so much more. We are beginning to understand epigenetics and the interaction of our genetics and lifestyle.

Nearly 20 years later, as I am diagnosed with these two new autoimmune diseases I looked back and I realized that I had Lupus for a long time, my first flare was in 1998, so I had had this disease for a very long time without a diagnosis. I looked at my life and I could see the cycles and the flares. I realized that this was different. This does not run in my family. This is autoimmune and I was told they come in packs.

I had changed my diet and my diet was healing my body. But I still had some serious work to do to understand these autoimmune diseases. I had learned enough about my body that I no longer believed that I was destined to my family's health history. I had turned back the clock. I felt better than I had felt in my entire adult life and yet I was diagnosed with a debilitating autoimmune disease. There were times when I couldn't get out of bed, when getting to the bathroom felt like it was a trek bigger than I could handle, when my whole body ached from head to toe. But those times were becoming less and less and for the first time in my life I had belief that I could beat this.

That was really when I went on a mission to cure Lupus. I had many medical experts, even those who practice alternative medicine and nutritional healing who gave me a bleak prognosis. They said I really wasn't going to be able to cure Lupus. "You're going to have to live with it. You're not going to be able to manage it. The best you can do is try to keep your symptoms under control with medications." The medications they wanted me to take; the steroids, the chemo medications, and the super antibiotics... I just said "no thank you" because I really believed that I was onto something. Nutrition and lifestyle played a much greater role than I had ever given it credit for. What I realized was that I thought I had a handle on my nutrition, and I did, but clearly it wasn't enough because I was still having flares.

So I took a look at my lifestyle. I took a look at that programming. I took a look at "Why is it that I don't listen to my body? Why is it that I need to work harder than I am physically able? Why do I do more than I am physically able?" I realized it was my programming. That is where I got my value. That is where I got my self-worth from. It's by being the best at what I do. It's by volunteering for the things that need to be done. It's by seeing more patients, taking on more caseload, or taking on more management and administrative responsibilities. That was how I got my value.

I would not slow down. I would not listen to my body and so it would shut down. It would attack itself. I realized that the first lesson Lupus taught me is that my genetics are not my destiny. My beliefs and programming run strong through family patterns. I can change that programming by the choices I make.

LESSON 2

Eat Your Fruits & Veggies

This may seem like a no brainer. This may seem pretty obvious. But when you are dealing with chronic pain you really don't value life. You really don't care. I didn't really care if I lived or I died. I do believe in God and I do believe in Eternal Life. To give up this life that I believed to be hard, painful, overwhelming and just quite frankly miserable, to be able to live with my Lord and Savior seemed so much better. I've never been afraid of death, and during that time in my life would have preferred to die rather than live.

I was in survival mode. I was on auto pilot and that is where life took me. I wasn't making any conscious choices. Well I was… but I was making them built on inaccurate beliefs; the limiting beliefs of fear and scarcity. I believed that life was a hard test and I was ready for the test to be over.

I had 3 children when I began this journey and I realized at that time that my perspective was selfish. Although I felt like death would be an easy answer to the pain and struggles in life, that choice was not fair to them (or my husband). I had lost my father to a massive heart attack when I was 16 and I realize now the impact that had on my life. I did not want to leave my children without a mother.

So understand that this was my mindset and my normal: Chronic pain from Rheumatoid Arthritis that I had learned to live with because doctors, mediations and therapies had not relieved it; wife and mother of 3; small business owner and operator. Like you, I did what needed to be done because it had to get done.

You've heard the saying that people change for 2 reasons; out of inspiration or desperation. I guess I'm an anomaly because I was too clueless for either! My change was by accident. In hindsight, it was all a perfectly orchestrated miracle by God but at the time it was just mind blowing.

I attended my regular Toastmasters group meeting and heard a presentation about a product that was fruits and vegetables in capsules. It was fascinating. I remember thinking, "WOW how cool is that?" but after the meeting I went back to work and honestly thought nothing more about it.

Until a couple of weeks later when at a Women's Health Care networking meeting I met another lady who gave a presentation on these same capsules. She shared the Children's Health Study with the group. My wheels started turning because I had been struggling with concerns of my daughter's diet. I thought "Well, this couldn't hurt and hers is free if I eat them too." So I signed up to eat the fruits and veggies every day with my daughter as part of the Children's Health Study for one year. I was hoping that the Juice Plus+ would fill whatever nutrient deficit she was having. I did not even consider a hopeful benefit of my own because I thought I was healthy!

Despite being overweight, exhausted, ordering pizza nearly nightly and eating out multiple meals a day on the run, chronically sick and chronically in pain…it was my normal. Nothing had changed my normal in the past 20 years, why would anything change it now?

Interestingly the timing for this "intervention" happened at the same time that I was approaching my 40th birthday and having the realization I talked about in Lesson 1. I was keenly aware that I was spiraling in a very bad direction based on my genetics and knew I had a bleak future if I didn't make some changes. I really couldn't bear the thought of exercise because I was in so much pain just functioning. I had my 10 vitamin regimen I took daily so my diet was ok, or so I thought.

I will never forget the day I was sitting at my desk after a long day of patients and charting. My hands didn't hurt! I couldn't remember the last time my hands didn't hurt. I literally looked at my hands and moved my fingers in awe. What had happened? I suddenly realized that I was experiencing the results of the antioxidants reversing the free radical damage and oxidative stress in my body. It had been about 6 weeks. I really didn't expect to feel much more than the improved energy from increasing my fruits and vegetable intake; after all I DID eat fruits and veg. I just didn't eat the variety, quantity and quality that the Juice Plus+ capsules gave me.

Mind blown! I became a full-on nutrition nerd. I had to learn how these fruits and vegetables in capsules had done what no doctor, therapy, or medicine had done in 20 years. I became obsessed learning about cellular health, nutritional healing, alternative healing, and holistic healing. I studied every book I could find. Practiced every type of healing I could research. I attended every class, workshop or conference that would expand my knowledge of rebuilding and supporting our bodies with nutrition.

The first thing I learned is that fruits, vegetables and berries are full of phytonutrients and plants are the only place you can get them. Why does this matter? Well because they are anti-oxidants. Why does this matter? Anti-oxidants neutralize the free-radicals that are damaging cells and creating oxidative stress. You cannot prevent oxidative stress. It is the byproduct of any oxygen consuming system.

Visualize a fire for a moment. As the fire burns it produces smoke. There is no way to have a fire without smoke. The larger the fire, the more smoke. Now it doesn't take a genius to know that smoke isn't good for you. The smoke is the byproduct of the energy produced by the fire. Heat or power is what you want but you cannot have either without the smoke. If I want to heat my home with a fireplace I need a chimney to direct the smoke outside where it can disperse. If the flue is closed and the smoke backs up in my home it can become deadly when enough of it accumulates.

Our bodies are like the fire. Every single minute of every single day that we are breathing oxygen and creating energy with our hearts beating we are creating "smoke" or oxidative stress by releasing the energy of life. If we workout we are building a bigger fire which, you guessed it, creates more smoke. The only way to eliminate your oxidative stress is to turn off your engine (die). Since that's not really the goal here we'll look for a better solution. Phytonutrients!

Here's an important kicker. Unlike smoke, we can't see or even feel oxidative stress in our bodies. Well, you can if you know what you are looking for but most of us just brush it off as aging. I am blessed because I have autoimmune diseases that let me know when my oxidative stress is accumulating. It shows up as pain in my joints, lesions on my skin, or even deep fatigue. Those are where I know my body stores oxidative stress.

Others are not as fortunate. Take my Dad for example. He did not have any awareness of the cardiac disease with arterial sclerosis and plaque that was building up in his arteries as a result of oxidative stress. Not until he had so much "smoke in the house" that it took his life, without warning. Unfortunately, my Dad's scenario is much more common than mine. Most people are completely unaware of the damage in their body or that they can "build a chimney".

So now we know WHY our moms told us to eat our veggies. Now we know WHY they are good for us. I would argue that they are not only good for us, they are essential. They provide a chimney, if you will, to haul out the smoke from our bodies before it has a chance to do any more damage. Is that enough?

This is where I became a self-proclaimed antioxidant junky. Remember I already mentioned that I had my 10 vitamin supplements that I took pretty faithfully. I also like fruits and veggies so they were a regular side dish to my dinner meal. I even had salads for lunches fairly regularly. Three more important lessons became apparent to me when I looked into why Juice Plus+ had relieved my pain.

1) Quality:

Isolated vitamins and supplements are not the same as eating whole foods. Yes, there may be some benefit from taking an isolated supplement for a short period of time but research has shown over and over that multivitamins do not work. Why? Because they are isolated and fragments of nutrients that we know help support the body. Many are synthetic, not even plant extracts. Yes, some are anti-oxidants but, when taken out of the plant based vehicle, the phytonutrient loses the thousands of compounds that scientists haven't yet isolated and put into the supplement with that vitamin. Man just can't replace what my husband calls "God's pharmacy".

Then there is the whole issue of the food industry. I am a gardener and have always had a garden except for the college years living in apartments and rentals. Maybe I should have been more aware of our food supply than I was. Again, I think I just took it for granted. I didn't really think about the fact that even in rural Idaho, most of our produce comes from Mexico and California. Most of it is commercially grown with herbicides and pesticides because we like our perfectly symmetrical blemish free produce at the supermarket. As a commercial grower, greater yields equals greater profits. Being treated and engineered to be more resistant to the transit process, packaging and shelf life has taken its toll on the quality of the nutrients in the foods we buy at the grocery store.

Produce must be picked before it is ripe so that it can ripen in transit. It just isn't viable to pick it ripe off the vine, package, transport, and finally put it on a shelf. Anyone who has had ripe berries or apricots or lettuce knows that if it is picked ripe you are lucky to have a few days in the house before it starts to rot. By the way, that is the sign of real whole food. It is natural for food to rot. If your food hasn't rotted any time recently you are eating "franken food" that has been modified.

2)   Quantity:

Again, as I took my 10 vitamin supplements, I chose them based on the support they were supposed to provide for my joint health, my heart health, and my brain health. Those were all systems that were not functioning well or that I was concerned about because of my family history. I was trying to identify the need and treat it, because that is what I do as a healthcare provider. Now I realize how silly it was for me to think that I knew better than God what nutrients my body needed to support and optimize my engine. God put all of the phytonutrients my body needs into whole foods. It isn't any more complicated than that. My body knows what to do with them. I just have to eat them.

Part of the problem is that the world we live in has fanned the flame of our fires and we have so many more toxins to haul out than ever before. Whether it's the external pollutants we ingest, breathe, or absorb through our skin; we see and feel it all around us.

Research studies now suggest consuming 10-13 servings of whole food produce daily, and don't forget the rainbow! Those foods need to be of different colors because each color has different anti-oxidant properties that support different systems of the body to maximize efficiency of your machine.

That was the secret. That was the reason Juice Plus+ had effectively hauled out the damage stored in my body that was presenting as pain. It was also the reason I had energy like a teenager. It was the reason I could release the weight that was protecting my cells from further damage. The reason I turned back my aging clock and looked like I was at least 10 years younger than my chronological years. My fountain of youth=anti-oxidant junky.

I was flooding my body with 30 different berries, vegetables, and fruits extracted from the whole raw foods vine ripened with all of the nutrients maintained. No pesticides, herbicides, or chemicals of any kind. No bacteria, fungus, or cross contamination of any kind. Juice Plus+ was cleaner, better quality and in a greater quantity than I was eating before.

3) Metabolic Programming

The really amazing thing that I was told about and understood logically was metabolic programming. You crave what you eat. I did recognize that if I eat more sugar, I crave more sugar. If I eat more salt, I crave more salt. Did you know that if you eat more plants you crave more plants?

We experienced that phenomenon in our family. After eating Juice Plus+ for a number of weeks, both my husband and son commented while we were out to dinner at a steakhouse that the broccoli was the best thing on the plate and they wanted more. WHAT? My husband and son, the meat eaters, wanted more broccoli? I was sure they had been abducted by aliens! It fueled my curiosity in and testimony of nutrition. It's true. When you eat more produce (Juice Plus+) you crave more produce (broccoli).

After nine years, our family, menus, cupboards, pantry and medicine cabinet look very different. It did not happen overnight but it was an early and powerful lesson that whole foods heal. That what we choose to put into our mouths matters. We now build our menus around the whole plants that are in season locally. We have much smaller portions of meat and dairy only occasionally.

Processed food is poison to my system and is one of the most rapid triggers to a flare so I try diligently to keep it out of my home and especially out of my mouth. We have not had an antibiotic prescribed for illness for anyone living at home since we changed our eating. This proves to me the power of healing with whole plant foods. Juice Plus+ broke the negative health cycle I was in and put me into a positive health cycle.

I do manage my health and my family's health by "doubling up" on my Juice Plus+ if I am going to be travelling, if I am around a lot of sick people, or if I am under particular emotional stress (good or bad). I know it can't hurt me and I have seen the effects of how it helps me, so I am quick to add a serving or two extra during that time to haul the toxins out and "get the extra smoke out" before it takes up residence and does damage.

We create new cells every single day, just like we create oxidative stress every single day. What do you want to feed those cells and what environment do you want to grow them in? I want my new cells to be as healthy and vibrant as possible as they replace my old damaged cells. When a patient tells me they are aching because they are getting old, I cringe. When my friends are taking statins, antidepressants, and antacids to deal with the effects of aging and life, I cringe. When patients and friends are taking injections and infusions of super-antibiotics and chemo therapy medications to manage their Lupus, I cringe. It's not immediate and some may even say it's hard, but I disagree. I think it is much harder to deal with the financial burden and lack of quality of life of my previous 20 years than the freedom and health of the last 9 years.

Rheumatoid Arthritis taught me the value of fruits and veggies. Lupus and Lichen Planus validated the research that I can heal my body through the choices I make. Juice Plus+ was the catalyst that restored my quality of life again. It gave me hope that I could build a better future for myself, my family and my community by inspiring healthy living, not only around the world, but starting under my own roof.

LESSON 3

Who Was I Born To Be?

As I went through my journey of healing, I was asked the question. "Who were you born to be?" I thought back to my childhood and my personality. I was very outgoing. Life was fun! I was very loud. I was the center of fun, the center of attention. I liked to have my friends around me. My world was all about having fun and being that catalyst for fun.

I realized that as I have grown I was often told, "Cally settle down" "Cally be quiet". Basically, that I was too much. I learned that I needed to be quieter. I needed to be calmer. I needed to not make such a big statement. Not have such a big presence. Now, as an adult, I looked at who I had become.

I had become a control freak. I became consumed with providing for my family and had high expectations that were never met. I was sabotaging my marriage by discounting my dependence on my husband. I was always feeling like I needed to be more responsible: make more money; have a bigger title. Getting that value from the world around me rather than recognizing my own value within me.

I went through a period of reflection (when you are sick you have some time to think). I decided that I had had a glimpse of health and I had had some reminders of who I used to be. So I went on a journey to remember who I was born to be.

Now I'm very passionate about helping people connect with that energy and their purpose. The reality is, I believe, we are all born with everything that we need to fulfill our life's mission. God equipped us with the personality, the energy, the temperament, the drive, that will get us through the challenges, the triumphs, and the opportunities that our life will bring to us.

I looked at this disconnect between who I was and who I was born to be. I had an "ah-ha moment". I realized, "of course I'm sick!" I was so out of balance. I was living such a lie. It wasn't bad. It was all good stuff. I'm a good person, but it was not true to me. It was not who I was born to be and so this misalignment between my purpose and my beliefs resulted in dis-ease.

I now refer to it as a misalignment between my spirit, my mind, and my body. Basically my spirit and my mind were at odds because my spirit had been told, by society and eventually by myself, to settle down and be quiet. My spirit knew better. My spirit knew what I was born to be because our spirit is eternal. It saw my mind limiting it, controlling it, dictating what it should be doing. What it should be doing did not feel right. I had a massive disconnect and imbalance with an internal struggle that became apparent. That internal struggle was manifest as a massive physical breakdown in my body. My body was literally attacking itself with autoimmune diseases.

When I reflected on the lesson Lupus taught me, the lesson was; "You are out of balance. You have forgotten who you were born to be. You were born to be fun. You were born to be a leader. You were born to be a teacher. You were born to help. You were born to create."

Well that's all well and good but we live in a world that believes you need to be responsible, you need to provide and you need to settle down. So I had to retrain my mind to trust my spirit, to have faith that I have everything I need to have. I don't have to be afraid of failure. I don't have to be afraid of scarcity. I don't have to have limiting beliefs that keep me in a safe little box. Those are lies. Those are lies that the world has put upon me. That my family has put upon me. That I have put upon me.

This isn't blame. It isn't an excuse. It's just a lesson that I've learned. I listen to my spirit. Remember who I was born to be. Be true to my gifts, and talents, and values. Trust my body. Know that my body can do the things that it needs to do.

My body was built to perform. It was built to create. It was built to exceed and excel, but not at the wrong things. If I have my focus in the wrong place, then I have that disconnect. If I have that disconnect, I have a flare because my body is out of balance and out of harmony; because I have forgotten who I was born to be and I am surviving with who I was taught to be.

I am loud and I do have high energy. I now recognize that it's ok to have fun. It's ok to do lots of things. It's ok to be a visionary. It's ok to dream. It's ok to make the world a better place. You don't have to make the world a better place by being someone else. You can be true to yourself. Lupus taught me to listen to my spirit. To remember who I was born to be. Because when I do that I'm in balance and harmony, and my body doesn't feel the need to attack itself to be heard.

LESSON 4

Health Is #1

I realize after being on the autoimmune rollercoaster that health is #1. Everybody has different priorities and I think for most people, and certainly I was one of those people, health was farther down the priority list. It may be number 3 or number 5. It follows making money to support your family. It certainly is secondary to your family. It may be secondary to your faith or God. It may be secondary to desires like food, leisure activities, and vacation. There is nothing wrong with any of those things and we all know that we have many priorities, interests and desires.

I believe that we are spiritual beings having an earthly experience. The reason we are here on earth is to be able to have experiences that we wouldn't be able to have as a spirit. We must have our physical bodies in order to do those things. You must have your health to do those things. If you don't then you can't fully experience those other things in the way you likely are intending to.

When you board a commercial airline, prior to your departure, you get the safety announcement. The airline attendant tells you how, in the event of an emergency, the oxygen mask will drop from above you and that you must put the oxygen mask on yourself before you put it on those minor children or dependent individuals who are travelling with you. You have to put your own oxygen on first! They also tell you that you may not see the bag inflate, but the oxygen is flowing.

This analogy rings true with the reprioritization of health that I was given with autoimmune challenges. If my oxygen isn't flowing, if I have not put on my own oxygen and I come into a crisis, I can't function. Life is a roller coaster. Life is an adventure. Life is a journey. We know that there are going to be unanticipated events whether they are exciting life changing events like birth and death and weddings and vacations or just routine things like change of seasons, aging, and work. These things all require your health.

I know the push back. I am familiar with the excuses and rationale. I had the same thoughts in the past. "I don't have time." "It's too expensive." "My kids come first." "My husband doesn't get it." I hear these comments all the time from people who have witnessed my transformation or need help reprioritizing in their own life. All I can say is that I've been there and that none of those perceptions are accurate. They are inaccurate perceptions. I'd like to address them by sharing my personal experience of each statement.

"I don't have time."

We all have the exact same amount of time in a day. 24 hours-- 1, 440 minutes-- 86,400 seconds. It is not how much time you have it is how you choose to use it. If you want to see where your true priorities lie, not your intention or lip service, look at your calendar. Appointments on your calendar are your true priorities because that is where you spend your time. Do you have mealtime on your calendar or do you squeeze it in or skip it? How about exercise? Sleep? Relaxation, entertainment, and socialization all impact your health or lack thereof.

I will be honest with you and tell you that I chronically struggle with "one more thing" and "I can do that" behaviors. I have had to consciously calendar the most important things into my schedule (my big rocks) so that they are the foundation of my year, month, week and day. If I don't put that structure into my calendar I will fall into the time-suck of the moment. I will go into this more in Lesson 5 but for now suffice it to say that I no longer use "I don't have time" as an excuse to not take care of myself.

"It's too expensive."

Again, if you want to know your financial priorities look at your bank statement. Where do you spend your money? The perception that nutritious food is expensive is absolutely false. It does not cost more to make a meal from whole ingredients than it does processed ingredients. Pre-packaged, convenience, frozen foods in the long run will always cost more than whole foods. There are a couple of reasons for this.

First, you eat less whole foods. I can sit down and eat an entire bag of potato chips without batting an eye, especially if I'm watching a show. Have you ever tried to sit down and eat 4 pounds of baked potatoes? What's the difference? The difference is the processing. You lose the nutrients and the bulk from the whole potato which nourish and satiate and replace it with fat and salt which sabotage digestion and addict the brain with metabolic programming. Remember you crave what you eat. Not only do you eat more of it, but your body has not been fed recognizable nutrients to use and so you are hungry again as your body searches for fuel.

Second, whole foods cost less, especially plant based whole foods. Again, going back to my potato analogy, today an average price for a Lays Potato Chip (my personal favorite) is 54.8 cents per OUNCE at Walmart. You can buy a 10 POUND bag of russet potatoes at that same Walmart for $1.94. Along the same lines I have never seen any produce that runs from $4.99 on average to $14.99 per pound; however, these are the prices that we pay every day for meat and dairy. This is especially the case with local and seasonal produce but holds up even with organic and specialty produce.

I know these two facts to be true because I saw the change in my monthly grocery bill when we switched from the Standard American Diet to a Whole Foods Plant Based Diet. When I use the term diet I am not speaking of the latest fad or weight loss program. I am referring to the foods you routinely eat for sustenance.

I changed my menu planning in two ways that reflected in my diet. First, I actually was intentional about what I ate so we had menus in addition to mealtimes. The focus for the menu planning became around what was seasonal in my garden, the farmers market or the produce section of the grocery store. Meat and dairy are not in every meal and they are never the focus of the meal. The standard in our house is getting it as close to the source as possible. If it comes out of a factory instead of a field it's not likely to make the cut.

When you eat whole foods you find you have fewer cravings. I still remember when I walked through my local Albertsons after work one day and had no problem getting the item I needed and checking out. This previously would have been a craving battle to not buy everything that jumped out at me and eat it while I was preparing dinner with the item I went in to get. I don't ever have that struggle now. I go in knowing exactly what I need and have no pull to the impulse items laid strategically along my path all the way in and out of the store to increase my grocery bill.

Our grocery bill was quickly cut in half when we changed our family's diet. Yes, I said family's diet because as the mother I set the example. I buy it and I cook it so they eat it. By putting MY oxygen on first by making my health #1 priority, I am now helping them reset their metabolic programming and cravings and ultimately health priorities as well. What they choose to eat outside of my house is up to them but at least at home they are nourished not just fed, and they now can feel the difference.

That is just the grocery cost side of things. It doesn't take an accountant to realize the cost savings of minimizing your health care costs. Our costs have plummeted here as well.

"My kids come first"

Maybe I addressed this in the previous paragraph. By taking care of yourself you are taking care of your kids. The reality is that if you do not take care of yourself you may not be there for your kids. I am a completely different mother now than I was before I revised my priorities. Yes, initially I felt selfish taking time for myself and certainly the whining about changing our diets was painful at first. It is so worth it now!

My youngest daughter has no recollection of my sick days. She will never know her mother as not being able to get out of bed and having to care for her. Fortunately, she was young enough when I changed my lifestyle that going for bike rides, 5 mile walks, and daily yoga are normal. That is not the mom that the older kids had. So while I may take more "selfish me time" than I used to, the quality of the time and amount of time I have for my family is drastically different and I think they would each tell you it is worth it.

Additionally, the health care experience and cost comparisons between my children are staggering. Both of my older children had serious seasonal allergies that shut them down for 6-8 weeks each spring. My oldest daughter was on prophylactic antibiotics from the age of 2 months – 8 years. My son was on daily nebulizer treatments from age 2-5 years. My youngest daughter has never been to the doctor except for well child checkups. She has never taken an antibiotic and rarely takes a pain reliever or allergy medication.

Our medicine cabinet which used to have all of the usual stomach remedies, pain relievers, allergy medications and prescription medications is unrecognizable. The cabinet now has band aids, coconut oil, essential oils, and Tylenol.

I didn't even recognize the change until my husband had his knee replacement surgery in 2014. As I stood there waiting for the pharmacist to fill the prescriptions from his discharge I was in awe as I wandered the aisles. I hadn't been in a pharmacy for so many years. It was so foreign and exciting that we hadn't been shopping these aisles.

Based on my experience, cost is the poorest excuse in the book. It just doesn't hold up. I have cut our grocery costs AND our health care costs SUBSTANTIALLY by making health #1. No matter how you slice it, a pound of prevention is cheaper than an ounce of cure!

By putting my health as #1 my kids (and grandkids) have a much different experience. I am able to participate in activities that I used to watch. I am more energetic and generally happier because I am not in chronic pain. I'll tell you that pain and fatigue can make the happiest person miserable and irritable. I am sure it was not fun being my child during that time. It wasn't fun being me! I'm still a work in process but at least I'm making progress as I've painfully learned these lessons.

"My husband doesn't get it"

I'm lucky. My husband has always been my #1 fan and will trust my judgment in whatever crazy idea I have. Don't think that means we always agree or that we are on the same page. We rarely are. However, it does mean that he will let me do what I want and, like the kids, he sees the benefits and eventually (pretty quickly in this case) jumps in whole heartedly.

I will take a minute here to brag on my husband. He has not only supported me in my lifestyle choices, but decided to come along with me. He added Juice Plus+ to his diet and noticed improved energy and very few colds. He has lived with chronic pain from a knee injury he experienced while serving in the US ARMY. In 2014, due to the ongoing bone on bone degeneration, pain and impact on his hip, back and ankles it was determined that he would be a candidate for a total knee replacement at age 45. He doubled up on his Juice Plus+ a month prior to surgery and during his recovery. His recovery was remarkable being able to go back to martial arts training in 2.5 months. Four months later, he was hiking the red rocks of Sedona, Arizona during a week's vacation with friends. He is now 3 years post-surgery and more active at 48 than he was at 38. He too has learned that health is priority #1.

Sometimes our husbands, children, even extended family don't have to "get it". They just have to allow you to "get it". Remember it's your choice, and you will have more influence than you know. The ripple effect of health priorities is so much lovelier than the whirlpool of pain and illness.

My lifestyle is just that, mine. I am the one who has to make the choice and I am the one who has to deal with the consequences. I cannot change anyone else, nor do I need to (more on that in Lesson 8). I realize as a wife and mother that I influence and have effect on my family but ultimately my choice is mine and their choice is theirs. I am blessed. My family does get it, though initially they were skeptical and there has been resistance here and there. They now see the value. The proof is in the quality of life.

Ownership and personal accountability for our health is critical. As a health care provider and a previous chronic health care patient, I truly believe that the only way we will ever reverse the epidemics and health care system cost and breakdowns is by staying out of the system. We stay out of the system by taking responsibility for our choices and lifestyles. Our healthcare system is equipped to fix acute problems such as broken bones and acute infections. It is not equipped to treat chronic disease. The primary reason is that most chronic diseases are a result of lifestyle choices. It is our culture to go to the doctor when we are sick and obtain a medication to treat that illness. We are not programmed to go to the doctor and ask what we should change in our lifestyle that may prevent us from getting the illness in the first place. We are reactive rather than proactive.

Medications are prescribed which create side effects which create the need for further medications and increases the risk of interactions. Medication management is a huge priority for health care providers because of the inherent risk. Even though I am a Speech Language Pathologist and do not prescribe or manage medications, I am required to ask my patients at EVERY visit if they have had any changes in their medications and reconcile that with their medical record and contact the primary care physician if anything flags as high risk or interaction risk. My average patient has 14 medications. Every time they come back from a hospital stay and often times even an ER visit, the medications have been changed. It is a tangled web we weave… You know what happens when you get caught in a web?

I am beginning to see a turning tide. More and more doctors are focusing on wellness and encouraging their patients to make lifestyle changes rather than just seeking medications. Unfortunately, it is not enough and that is because it needs to start with us. It starts with me. If I make the choice to change my health priority, I in turn change my health story which in turn changes my health history which in turn changes my family's health history. If you choose to do the same thing, we start to see momentum in the community which begins to change the culture of the community and the expectations as we go to our wellness providers (which many doctors would love to be) rather than our sick care providers (which many doctors are frustrated as). Making health priority #1 rather than expecting a magic pill will go a long way in improving the dysfunction of our health care system. In the end, it is up to me, not a doctor, not a system, not an insurance company what my health is. Reality is a bitter pill to swallow.

This is why I say health is #1 priority, because if you are in a hospital it doesn't matter who you need to see on the docket today. It doesn't matter what is in your inbox at work. It doesn't matter who is depending on you to be at a meeting. If you are incapacitated because of an injury or an illness and you don't have your health for that period of time. Nothing else matters. You can't go to the games with your kids. You can't participate in the family event. You can't go on vacation. You can't earn income. You can't fulfill your responsibilities and obligations if you don't have your health.

That is why health became my #1 priority. As my health took the focus that was required, it took a lot of focus and a lot of prioritization in the beginning to get my health back, to reclaim it. I should mention it still takes conscious mindful choice-making to sustain it.

I must continue to make mindful choices about the food I put in my body and the exercise I use to maintain my strength and vitality. I must be mindful of the stress I am putting myself into that is taxing my chemical production of cortisol and adrenaline burning out my adrenal system. I must be mindful of the free radical damage and oxidative stress in my body, putting in the antioxidants to offset the damage that I am doing just by living every day. I need to be realizing that "hey, I'm under more stress" or "hey, I'm around a lot of sick people right now" or "hey, I'm not getting to bed on time" so I need more antioxidants. I need to change what is going in my mouth and increase my antioxidant intake.

This is a lesson that Lupus taught me, health is #1. If your health is limiting your choices that you can make in your life, it doesn't matter how much money you have. It doesn't matter how much time you have. It doesn't matter how many relationships you have. It matters that you can't participate in those relationships, in those activities that you earned the money for or the time that you have taken.

Really you have a lot of time when you are sick, because you can't do anything, basically you are just healing. You have to put your health as #1 priority and not feel guilty. It is necessary and it is critical that you take time to take care of yourself and that you are aware of your health and making it priority #1 so that you can use that body to experience all of the wonders you were created for.

LESSON 5

Empty Your Cup

This is actually a lesson that comes from Bruce Lee that my husband teaches in his martial arts. You empty your cup of knowledge so that you can take more in. If you are so sure that your way is the right way or the only way or that you are an expert and don't need to learn anymore; your cup is full and you are not able, or should I say willing, to learn more knowledge.

I have found that this applies in two ways for me in living with autoimmune disorders. First, I've learned to open my mind to many types of healing and to learn something from each of them. Second, I've learned that it's important to empty my cup daily to touch base with my mind and my spirit so that I am connecting my body and allowing new knowledge to fill my cup.

When the student is ready the teacher will appear. I have heard that statement several times in my life and it certainly is true, although as with most of these lessons, I didn't realize it at the time.

Just shortly after the now infamous 40th birthday, and my new-found obsession with all things nutritional healing, I met another lady at the same women's health networking group. She had recently completed schooling for Ama Bodywork and was offering a complimentary massage to increase understanding of Ama Bodywork and help grow her practice. Up to that point in my life, I had been to a few massages but I was a novice to say the least.

I remember that lying on my stomach was pretty much impossible at that time. It certainly was not comfortable. Immediately Ama was different because she had me lay on my back, felt my radial pulses and checked my tongue. This, of course, peaked my interest because I am a speech therapist so I know a little something about tongues! I did not know that you could tell how my organs were functioning and where my stress was piling up by assessing my tongue and pulses. Fascinating!

She probably just wanted me to be quiet and experience the Bodywork, but I was so intrigued with Ama that it was a constant barrage of questions the entire hour. I scheduled another appointment and another and another soaking up the therapy that was amazing as well as the Traditional Chinese Medicine philosophies that it comes from. For a period of about 3 years, I had Ama Bodywork regularly, until she closed her practice to stay home with her children and I eventually moved. What I learned during that time, during what I dubbed "massage with a purpose", continues to fill my cup to this day.

This is where I first learned about the meridians and chi. In my mind, Ama is similar to acupuncture as it uses points along the meridians to release pain, blocks and dysfunction although Ama Bodywork uses acupressure or massage. An acupuncturist can identify a problem and put a needle into a specific point to relieve the problem, similarly my Ama therapist would assess and determine what meridian was in most need and work on it. Fire cupping and stones were my favorite way to get rid of incredible knots!

It is still incredible to me when I look back on that time and all that she moved out of my body. At that time I did not have the understanding of my own body and systems to effectively move the toxicity that had been building up for years. Without really understanding it I was on a toxic overload overhaul. I will be forever grateful for my empty cup that was continually filled as I changed my scientific, allopathic/western medicine, disease care, symptom treatment approach to a holistic medicine, health focus, cause prevention approach to my life and practice.

You can probably guess that this opened up another voracious appetite for learning all that I could about alternative healing beginning with Traditional Chinese Medicine, Reflexology, the 12 meridians and yoga. I was learning how all of this related to nutrition and nutritional healing as I was introduced to the impact of eating for the seasons. How foods support our organ function and vary according to the season. What has more recently grown in acceptance and popularity as eating what is in season and grown locally.

As I look back on my initial Ama Bodywork, it was critical as a preparatory phase to my understanding of my body. At that time, I only knew of the Rheumatoid Arthritis and I certainly didn't consider it an autoimmune disorder. Allopathic or Western Medicine didn't label it as such back then. It was classified a degenerative disease.

My Ama therapist would assess my meridians and organ function. I was always low in spleen, lung, or liver. She would move out the toxins and strengthen those systems and teach me foods, herbs and cooking techniques that would support my systems. I felt more and more amazing over time.

This was the point I was at when I received the diagnoses of Lupus and Lichen Planus. This was part of the reason I had faith in my body and my ability to heal if I could just give it the right environment to do so. I had some knowledge but I did not have the tools to effectively finish what I started, so I continued.

I know that it was a tender mercy of my Father in Heaven to withhold my autoimmune diagnoses until I had found this knowledge. I truly believe that if I had received this diagnosis 3 years earlier, prior to my nutritional healing and holistic healing knowledge, I would have taken the medications and treatments prescribed by my trio of doctors, I would have resigned to the pain and misery, and I would likely not be alive today. I certainly would not be ALIVE today!

For a time, I actually left healthcare because it was so toxic. I just didn't have the tools or understanding at that time to recognize what I was picking up and carrying around with me all the time. My systems were so blown out and depleted it took years to rebuild them.

I continued to empty and fill my cup expanding my study to the chakras which led me to the fascinating field of energy work. This was what I now recognize as the missing piece in my total transformation. I still don't have the skill that my Ama therapists have at being able to assess my system and address it relating a specific point on a specific meridian to a specific organ or muscle group. However, I do now understand the relationship of the energetic body to the physical body.

Initially I think part of my closed mind or fear of energy work came from the perception of mysticism. I come from a traditional Christian background with a strong belief in God the Father, His Son Jesus Christ and the Holy Spirit. I pray to God through and in the name of Jesus Christ to thank him for my blessings, and to ask for blessings of strength and healing. Somehow connecting with "energy" on my own was maybe sacrilegious or blasphemous.

Referring to Universe was discounting my belief and recognition of God. Though this may be the case for some who do not believe in God and feel only a connection to the universe and mankind in general, I have found that it really has nothing to do with energy work.

Quite the contrary, I have found that understanding my connection to my energetic self, my mind and spirit, has strengthened my personal connection with God. I feel so blessed that He has gifted this knowledge to me so that I may use it and share it to improve my life and the life of those around me.

I really grasped the concept of our energy system when I looked to our Western medicine diagnostic testing that I am personally familiar with, the EKG and the EEG, even the imaging diagnostics Ultrasound, CT Scans, MRI Scans, and PET Scans. None of these diagnostics are looking at microorganisms under a microscope or even looking at blood or serum samples. There is very little "physical" analysis done. What all of these tests use is ENERGETIC testing. They measure the heart or brain function not by physically putting a port to your heart or brain but rather through an electrode that measures your energetic function through physical manifestations. Similarly, the imaging tests are completed by holding an imaging sensor across the area of concern or even more removed, having you lie in a machine not even touching you, to have the imaging sensor read your energy and create a picture of your physical organ or area of concern.

The kicker is that we do not yet have the technology to measure and read ALL of the different types of energies around us and in our bodies. Because of this we are slow to recognize what we don't see or understand. At least I know I am…

All you have to do is look at technology and the reality of today's cell phones. The amazing capabilities that are being realized sending complex documents, pictures, or movies out into a cloud that you can somehow put an address on and retrieve on demand in an instance from anywhere at any time. I now realize that not believing in an energetic system and its connectedness with everyone everywhere would be similar to thinking the world is flat or living in a cave. It's primitive thinking.

As my exposure to energy work expanded, I learned of Tapping. It is an amazing technique that can be done by anyone, anywhere, at pretty much anytime. Tapping was easy and familiar to me because of the foundational knowledge I had of the meridians. It was so effective at clearing energy blocks and toxins I was blown away. The coolest thing was that it was a physical tool much like Ama that I could use myself, even with my limited understanding of the energetic system.

I now have a plethora of effective techniques and tools that clean and clear my energetic system. I now understand that I pick up energies throughout my day living my life much like the oxidative stress that happens inside my physical body. Some of those energies are toxins from the energy pollution of technology all around us that overstimulates and confuses our personal energy fields. Much like the feedback you get when the mic is too close to the speaker or when you are losing range of a radio station or you have crossover frequencies because you are traveling between regions.

Some of the energies are from people or circumstances I encounter throughout the day. Some of the energies have been passed on to me through my family just like my physical characteristics are passed on through my DNA physical structure. Some of these energies are amazing like love and peace others like fear and pain are not so welcome.

Just like I wouldn't go weeks without a shower and eating nutritious food I now wouldn't think of going weeks without energy clearing and thinking supportive thoughts. "Garbage in, garbage out" used to be an adage I used for junk food but I will tell you that we have an even bigger problem with junk thoughts and the damage is so much harder to release. It takes daily energy hygiene, just like daily physical hygiene to keep my body vital and prime.

Lupus has taught me to empty my cup daily and to fill it daily. The lessons of this life are meant to be learned and applied so that we can progress into a fuller and more meaningful purpose and experience. If we get stuck in the past or focus on the future we miss what really matters today. I have learned to be intentional in all that I do but not a know-it-all or control freak. I have learned to dream and aspire but not wish and worry. Maybe most importantly, I have learned to be grateful for my past and learn from it but not have regrets or re-dos.

This lesson is still in progress. As I mentioned, I still have a great deal to learn and understand about the energetic part of my body, but I love it and have learned to respect it and value the messages and interaction it has with my physical body. I am grateful now for my autoimmune diseases because they give me a physical warning that something is off with my energy. I now recognize the warning signs and do not have to be incapacitated to recognize that I am out of sync. Best of all, I now have tools to be able to not only recognize it but also manage it. For me, it is the best prevention I know to date.

LESSON 6

How Do You Eat
An Elephant?

My personality and wiring was such that I needed to do everything. Do it all myself. Do it all now! There was a great sense of urgency and to me that was just normal. It wasn't until my sister pointed this out to me that I realized it wasn't normal for everyone.

My sister is quite a bit older than I am, in fact 15 years older. We are essentially from two different generations. She is a baby boomer. I am a Gen Xer. That's just how our lives have been… different. She has been a great support and help to me throughout my life, but really more of a mother figure rather than a sister figure because of our age difference and birth order.

In 1998, she had gone back to college and was writing a paper. She needed to do an interview for this assignment so she called me and asked if she could come over and do an interview. When she came over, this is the scenario she encountered and described in her paper.

> She approached the door with the Halloween mat
> going off, the house fully decorated, cookies in the

oven and dinner being prepared. The kids were doing their activities and I had just gotten home from work. Quite frankly it was a pretty typical evening in our home.

During the interview she asked me why I live every day like it's my last and why I'm so driven. I said to her "What do you mean? Why do I...?"

I started to reflect and look around me. I had never, really, given any thought to my lifestyle. I was the first in my family to go on to college and just happened to choose a field that required a master's degree as the entry level education. I had never considered not going to college. I had watched my mom struggle to provide for us after my dad passed away. I also had begun working at that time for a regular paycheck to help ends meet. I knew that I needed to have a skill that would provide a reliable income so that, if I ever needed to, I would be able to provide for myself and my family.

Having a husband and children was the natural progression of life. I couldn't have thought about putting those off while I finished my education or choosing to have a career instead of a family. It's just not in my wiring. I couldn't imagine picking just one or doing just one step at a time because to me it seemed URGENT. I had to do it all. Doing less just wasn't an option.

I never took time. Never! Between the ages of 20 and 40, I have no recollection at all of scaling down or consciously choosing to put my health as a priority. I was very much in survival mode. I was very much on autopilot. I had no awareness whatsoever of the impact of the decisions I was making. I've never smoked. I never drank. I was not an athlete but I was busy. I never really worked out. I ate well. In fact, being busy and having a lot of food around me was almost "proof" that I was successful.

As I look back on that period of my life, it was not until I had the encounter with fruits and vegetables that literally changed my world. That encounter started me on the education of how antioxidants heal at the cellular level and how our lifestyle can either support that healing or sabotage that healing. I developed an understanding that I needed to delegate, I needed to prioritize, and I needed to slow down.

I realize now that not everybody operates like that. It's not an "ah-ha moment" for everyone. Things can be paced. They don't all have to be done now and you can delegate. You don't have to be everything. As I progressed through living with autoimmune diseases, I gave up perfection. I realized that I strive for excellence because perfection is exhausting and unattainable.

That was the first step. Then I started to realize that not only do I not need to be perfect, but I don't need to do it all. Delegation and prioritization came into my vocabulary. It just hadn't before. I just did it because it needed to be done. I got my value and self-worth from my list of accomplishments and how many to-dos I could check off in a day.

With the absolute shear exhaustion that comes with autoimmune flare ups and the incapacitating fatigue, I started to realize that I could prioritize and I could delegate. This understanding became central to managing my health.

Things still need to get done. I still have an ongoing list that I cross things off and I add things to. I still get a great deal of satisfaction in crossing things off my list. I add things to it so that I don't let them slip off my radar. However, it no longer has the urgency that it used to.

It truly is a prioritization. I look at my TOP 3 priorities each day. I pick three things! Any more than three is not realistic. The top priorities will get done. The other lessor to-dos will get done because they support the top priority, sub-steps, and will get done as you do priority #1. Some may fall off because they are not important or they will be delegated to someone who is able to do it. It may not be necessary for you to do it. There may be someone who is better suited to do it than you are.

I have taken this habit and refined it even more with 1 priority for me, 1 priority for my family, and 1 priority for work. Does that make you cringe to think I only do 3 things in a day? It would have made me crazy to think that way before this lesson was learned. Before my feet hit the ground in the morning I take a minute to reflect on what my 3 priorities are for the day. What will I do for me, my family and my work? Many other things come in and go out of the day but 95% of the time those priorities are not compromised and they get done.

I knew I had mastered this habit and turned over a new leaf when I was in a committee meeting at the University several years back. I sat around the conference table representing the department for an event we were participating in and co-sponsoring. We were providing space for the medical screenings, students to complete the screenings, and supervisors to oversee the organization and flow of the participants. As the event was planned and assignments were made I was able to effectively delegate tasks to the appropriate person to best manage each aspect of the event. The outside community representative looked at me and commented about my skilled delegation.

Much like my sister's observation and comment, his observation and comment resonated so strongly because I was no longer the leader that volunteered to do everything. I knew my strengths and priorities. I also knew the strengths and needs of the other team members or those who were not necessarily around the table. I knew who had something to contribute to the event that would be more valuable if they had ownership of it.

This was a skill I had been working hard to develop and it had been recognized by someone who had no idea of the mountain I had climbed to get there. He had given me a compliment that validated a mastery of excellence not perfection, of delegation not control.

There are far more shared tasks around our house than there used to be. I ask for help a lot more than I used to ask. I no longer feel inadequate or guilty if I can't accomplish something. I no longer feel guilty if I have to ask for help because that is all a part of taking the bites of the elephant. I'm not trying to do everything. I'm not being all things to all people. I still want to be a lot of things to many people but I realize that it's not necessary for me to live with that mock-10-hair-on-fire that I did for so many years absolutely on autopilot. I had no real awareness that I was completely and totally burning out my adrenal system because I was constantly running on adrenaline. I was constantly running in stress.

Still even saying "slow down" feels a little derogatory. It feels limiting. It feels like I'm not keeping up and doing everything I should do. But the realities of "slow down to speed up" or "less is more" sayings are true. For so many years, I heard these sayings but I couldn't understand them. I didn't internalize them. I didn't understand how the activities I choose to participate in affect my overall health and well-being. It's the difference between a flare and vitality.

As hard as I try, it still frustrates me because life still happens and it still triggers stress; but the difference is, I now look at the situation. I don't just run headlong into it. I now realize what I can and cannot control. What I need to control or not control in order to prioritize and delegate.

Lupus has taught me to look at and realize the elephant and recognize what bite will make the biggest impact for me. How do you eat an elephant? One intentional bite at a time!

LESSON 7

The Chrysalis Period

I use the butterfly to symbolize the transformation in my coaching practice. For me the butterfly is symbolic of transformation. As I selected the butterfly for symbolism, I still felt very much felt like a caterpillar surviving, going around munching on leaves and crawling on the ground, literally just trying to survive.

That period with my autoimmune diagnoses when I realized what I was dealing with and that the strategies that I had employed throughout my life for survival were in fact sabotaging me and making my health worse. That is when I realized that I needed to do something differently. That was the beginning of my chrysalis experience; when I went into a great deal of study of nutrition and of mindfulness, alternative healing with energy work, meditation, and spirituality with my Father in Heaven. I was digging deep into all the aspects of my life because my physical challenges created an opportunity for me to study and immerse myself in all the different aspects of my life; physical, mental and spiritual.

As I did that, I had my chrysalis experience over a five-year time span where I really enrobed myself in that focus and the change happened. As I learned all of those pieces of information, I applied it and often times it was still very much a struggle and felt very unnatural and challenging for me to apply some of these principles. They were very contrary to our Standard American Diet, very contrary to our Standard American Lifestyle, very contrary to my upbringing and belief systems. The tapes that I ran in my head and the beliefs that I had in my mind were uncomfortable to come up against and challenge them and reprogram my lifestyle.

My background is in neurocognitive rehab and retraining the brain. I have done that for 25 years but I didn't really grasp the relationship to my lifestyle. I related it to recovering from a brain injury or a stroke, some sort of neurological incident.

I would tell my patients, "3 things you must have for the best recovery; good mood, good food, and rest". That counsel came from my observation of patients who had a missing piece to that puzzle that would stall out their recovery. If I observed a weak area for the patient we would address it head-on with strategies to improve their mood, food, or rest and weave it into therapy to maximize their progress and outcomes. I didn't necessarily relate it to MY lifestyle.

It was both overwhelming and encouraging because I knew the results. I knew that neuro reprogramming was possible and that is basically what I was doing. I knew from experience that it wasn't a magic bullet. Change and progress requires a lot of practice and repetition. I was doing it throughout my entire lifestyle. It was a behavioral change, mindset change, brain change, chemistry change and it took place over that five-year chrysalis period.

Then in the last 1-3 years, I felt the awakening out of that chrysalis. I've been able to spread my wings as a butterfly. Even awakening into the new transformed butterfly took time. I felt like I would get a wing out and find myself in a flare and frustrated thinking "I thought I was past this."

The perfect example of this was when I decided to return to practice as a speech therapist two years ago. My favorite setting for rehab is home health because that is where you can really get to know not only the patients, but their families and support system. It's the most "real" environment for health care and it is so rewarding. It is also very flexible and low stress in comparison to other health care settings.

I had heard of a new company in the area whose therapy approach and culture closely aligned with mine. I was offered what seemed like a perfect position with full time pay and benefits at 32 hours a week with a company I was really excited to work with. Less than a month back in health care…bam…I was right back into old habits! Probably the most shocking to me was the mindless eating and hitting the drive-thru.

In my caterpillar life, it was very common for me to put whatever was in front of me in my mouth. When you are in home health and running between patients it is most convenient to hit the drive-thru. You have to stop and use the restroom anyway so why not grab something to eat as well? I work through meals often because I am evaluating the swallowing function of a patient and will miss my own meal.

At the University I had learned to pass on the massive amounts of junk food that was used as reward, marketing, and entertainment because I would fuel my body. I was very mindful of the choices I made. I could easily participate in any activity and had mastered my eating. At home I had complete control of my environment and schedule. I was shocked when I found myself back in the old triggers with the exact same autopilot behaviors surfacing.

Within a month of being back in health care, I was back in autoimmune flares that fluctuated in length and severity for the next

18 months. Despite recognizing the supportive habits and behaviors that my transforming butterfly was experiencing, I definitely had growing pains coming out of that cocoon and spreading my wings fully.

The difference this time around was much like my initial experience when I first felt no pain and increased energy after 20 years of being a caterpillar. I knew how good it felt to feel good! I couldn't go back to pain and depletion as "normal". I know how to heal and support my body. That has been my experience of transformation. I had felt the wings of the butterfly. I've come too far to go back.

So I continued, I will admit, with a great deal of frustration. I had to set up new strategies and triggers to be mindful and intentional. I had to refine and practice even more reprogramming. I would do great…and then fall back…until finally, the butterfly emerged.

I literally feel like I am thriving. I am flying. I am this butterfly who has now been freed of these autoimmune diseases. Not because they are cured but because I've been transformed by them. My lifestyle now supports my health instead of feeling trapped by my health.

I no longer need to use my health as an excuse or as a justification for me to slow down or for me to set boundaries. I now align with who I was born to be and use that as my justification rather than my health or lack thereof. My environment no longer defines me or triggers me because I define my environment. I choose my perspective and focus on how I respond to the things that are outside of my control. I am mindful of what I allow into my mouth, my mind, and my heart. I am 100% responsible for the choices I make and the resulting outcomes, good or bad.

I have gone through this transformation journey from the caterpillar surviving with a limited view and struggling lifestyle even though I had great abundance around me! Look at everything that is around the caterpillar. Everything is bounteous and plentiful and the caterpillar is by no means in threat of starvation or working too hard but yet that is how the caterpillar feels...munch, munch, munch.

The caterpillar then enters into the immersion period of the chrysalis with transformative learning and nurturing eventually awakening into a transformed state. Even in that transformed state as a butterfly that is now able to see the big picture and has a completely different view point of the world. The perspective is so grand and the hope and the joy and the peace are so great.

I always said that I would know when my transformation was complete because it would no longer be the exception to do these things, like meditation or eating a healthy diet. Making the healthy choice would just be making the choice versus good and bad. It would just be my normal. Some of my old behaviors would actually be the uncommon behavior. I have reached that point so I do know that my transformation has occurred and that I've emerged as the butterfly.

Even as the butterfly, you still land. You still land on the leaf. It's higher so that you have that different perspective, but you still have to rest. You still have to take it in. You can't fly all the time. You can't glory all the time. You can't just take it in and look around. Sometimes you have to sit and rest. Sometimes you have to nourish and continue that lifestyle and awareness that got you there in the first place because you can still get eaten by a bird or get squished as a butterfly.

It's not all glorious. I'm not cured of my autoimmune diseases. They are not gone. This is a journey and as my transformation journey has come into its fullness I recognize that it continues to be ongoing. It is not a destination that you reach and then you are done. Rather it continues to be something that you maintain and that you continue to grow. You continue to find new heights and new opportunities and in that you rest and restore. As you do those things, it supports the heights. That is a lesson that I continue to learn and continue to refine today.

LESSON 8

All You Need Is (Unconditional) Love

I've always been a caregiver type of personality. Maybe I get that from my mom. I've always been one that can relate to people and have a genuine empathy. My experience with autoimmune disease has given me a different understanding of compassion. I feel like I understand more than I did before of how important *unconditional* love is.

I now see that there was some selfishness in love, because I got validation out of caring for people. I got validation from my patients. It makes you feel good to help people and be a facilitator of improving their quality of life.

At home, I often had a reciprocal love from family. I do something for you, you love me. You do something for me, I love you. It of course wasn't intentional. I never thought that, I never felt "conditional". However, as I learned these lessons and did some deep dives into self-reflection, I recognized that I was guilty of building walls and holding hostages.

The autoimmune diseases made my weaknesses glaringly apparent to me. I initially was very angry and felt betrayed by my body. I hadn't "abused" my body. Why did it let me down? Why did it turn on itself? Why was it attacking innocent organs that were vital to its survival? I couldn't understand why I deserved this.

At some point in this journey I realized that my weaknesses were not only physical but they were emotional as well. I can't really pinpoint one event or particular ah-ha moment that this lesson occurred but rather a series of reflection, personal development, and spiritual growth that has made it clear to me.

Even now as I reflect on how to articulate this lesson it is difficult for me; maybe because it is the most personal, maybe because it is the most important, maybe because I am still refining.

As I reflect, I think I first learned this lesson very close to home in my marriage. I know I am the ONLY person who has ever been frustrated by a spouse. Why doesn't mind telepathy come with marriage vows? All kidding aside, as I look back on my behavior now it seems so ridiculous to me, although sometimes I still catch myself thinking or feeling some of those same feelings.

My husband and I come from different family structures and backgrounds. I am the youngest of 4 children raised on a farm by both of my parents across the state from my extended family. My husband is the older of 2 children raised in a small city by his mom with a great deal of involvement from his maternal grandparents. His dad was involved in his life on summers and holidays. His sister was born when he was 10 and grew up with her father in the home until he was in junior high school. He joined the military after graduating from high school when I went off to college.

That is where our worlds intersected. We were two people from completely different backgrounds who accidentally fell in love out of friendship and decided it would be a good idea to get married.

Very similar to the physical pain and stress of my 20s and 30s, I put that same emotional pain and stress on my marriage. Not intentionally. In fact, I was quite well intended in my crusade to "fix" my husband. I wanted to make up for all of the areas he felt neglected or abandoned. I wanted to make up for all of his inadequacies or insecurities. The only problem was that in doing so I completely disregarded his role as the patriarch of our family, the leader, the father, the provider. I made him feel even more inadequate, insecure, neglected and abandoned.

It was not until our marriage nearly fell apart for the third time that I finally got it! I was the one that needed to be "fixed". I was the only thing I could change. I brought my own insecurities, fears, loss, and inadequacies to this equation and I needed to look inside and identify what I wanted to change in ME not my husband.

Of course the most perfect examples of unconditional love come from our Father in Heaven and our Savior Jesus Christ. There are 389 references in the scriptures to love "as I have loved you". Although I heard it, read it, and knew it, I didn't do it.

I realized that I had to start with me so I took note of all the places I was falling short. Let me tell you, it is humbling and easy to turn into self-punishment as you beat yourself up for all of the things you have done to mess up the lives of those you care most about.

Fortunately, I continued to be taught this lesson of forgiveness and not only did it start with me, but I needed to forgive myself. I had to learn to love and accept myself. Not just lip service but truly love myself in spite of my imperfections. This included my body that I was very angry and frustrated by because it had betrayed me. I had to unconditionally love ME. That was hard because I didn't really know how.

Learning to forgive and love myself, as I am, with all of my faults and weaknesses was the most difficult project I've ever had in my life. It could only be done with the divine love from above. Feeling that acceptance, love, and worthiness came as I remembered who I was born to be. When I remembered that I am a daughter of God, and He created a being with potential to be exactly what I needed to be.

I was born with the innate character I would need to learn and grow with a body that would physically support me as was needed. My job here was to learn to love ME, not resent me or put me down for not being perfect. That is the destination, this is the journey. I came to know that when I am self-deprecating I am insulting God, discounting his creation and doubting my potential.

Once I finally came to love myself and truly understand what unconditional love meant, I found it easier to follow the commandment found in John 13:34 "A new commandment I give unto you, that ye love one another; as I have loved you, that ye also love one another." I have probably heard that scripture quoted hundreds of times since I was 3 years old and I am astonished that it took me so long to really understand it.

I was raised to be the end of gossip. I tried to be careful to not judge others. I always wondered why we treat strangers more kindly than we do our families. We speak more compassion at work than we do at home. Just like with my physical body, I thought I was doing ok; and it wasn't until I truly understood the joy and peace of unconditional love that I realized I could do so much better.

Enter 100% accountability. I cannot change or fix anyone, nor do I need to. That is their journey, your journey, not mine. What I have found, as I now look at my life through a different perspective, is that I am responsible for how I react to a situation. Am I frustrated because I had an expectation that they were going to do something and they didn't? They probably didn't even know I had that expectation. Am I carrying resentment because of the way I was treated? What did I do to put myself in a situation to be treated that way? What condition did I put on that person that qualified my love for them? If you…, then I ….

When I was truly honest with myself, I found that pattern rampant in my life. Criticism, blame, shame, guilt, complaint all took the responsibility off of me and put it on others. I realize that is not accurate and it certainly isn't love.

I found that when I released criticism, blame, shame, guilt, complaint and owned my reaction of acceptance, benefit of the doubt, compassion, forgiveness, and compliments I generally end up with a different end result. It certainly feels more like love.

It is different to love individuals where they are at, as they are, and not put my expectations on them. I find people let me down. Their priorities or interests or beliefs aren't necessarily in line with mine. It's not that they are intentionally letting me down. Realistically, they often don't even know my desires or expectations.

If I'm building my expectations, I'm having conditional love; even though I don't think I ever intended to have conditional love. I now realize that when you have expectations of someone (and that includes yourself), but your love, empathy, and compassion is not contingent upon that you don't hold them hostage or guilt them into your path.

I am not saying you shouldn't have expectations. I am one for setting a high bar, because I believe people will rise to whatever level you expect of them. I am saying that I need to have love for everyone, regardless of expectations.

Sometimes I still find myself falling short, but I feel that living with autoimmune diseases has blessed me to understand limitations; when you truly cannot get out of bed, when you truly have chronic pain, when you are angry and frustrated because you feel like your body has let you down. I think having some of those emotions and experiences has given me more gratitude and more selflessness to love others where they are, accept people with whatever limitations they have, and give grace for doing the best you can. Honestly that is all any of us can do.

I'm not perfect and although I haven't expected other people to be perfect maybe in their perception it came across that way. I feel like I have a new depth of love and compassion that is more genuine and unconditional than I had prior to my experience with Lupus.

It's true that you can't take it with you! Stuff, things, expectations don't matter in the end because what you have is love and your relationship regardless of your health, your wealth, your priorities. Living with autoimmune diseases taught me to love unconditionally because in the end that really is all you have.

Closing Thoughts

What I have learned on this journey is that our bodies are amazing and that two thirds of our life is not tangible. Two thirds of our body's existence and experience is not visible. We must tune in and recognize and maintain our mind and our spirit just as much as our body.

My body is my barometer that lets me know how well I am doing at caring for my mind and spirit in addition to my body. I now look at my autoimmune diseases as a blessing. They help me recognize and get my lifestyle choices back into check before I am too out of balance.

Daily meditation, prayer, and energy work along with recognizing and being just as aware of what I put in my mind as I am what I put in my mouth are critical. I now recognize that toxins are not only in our physical environment but also in our energetic environment and the world that we live in. It is my responsibility to take care of the gift that I have been given in my physical experience and to respect the mind and the spirit as well.

I believe that at the end of this life when my body is spent, that my mind and spirit will live on eternally. I believe that I will take with me all of the adventures, experiences and lessons that I have learned in this mortal life.

This time is so short and so precious. It's not about how long I live but how well I live. I now have that understanding. I now have a daily routine and practice. I now have transformed and believe that I will live a much longer life.

I think back to when I did not expect to live a long life at all, and in fact, did not want to live a long life because I was just surviving. Life was a difficult test that I wanted to be over. My perspective has changed. My life is now a wonderful adventure with many twists and turns, obstacles and opportunities, mountains to climb and vistas to take in. Now that I am thriving, I hope to live and expect to live well into my 100s. I am no longer bound by the Standard American Lifestyle, the Standard American Diet and my small life, small thinking. I am guided by my divine nature, by my eternal potential and an eternal perspective.

I am blessed to be thriving with Autoimmune Diseases. These were important lessons for me to learn and I hope that they in some way can touch your life or be the insight you were looking for on your journey. Hope, peace, joy and love were not what I found online when I googled Lupus but that is what I have found in my autoimmune journey. May you have similar findings on your journey.

About the Author

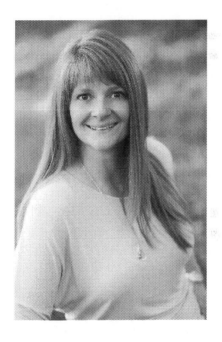

CallyRae is best known for her professional accomplishments as a Speech Language Pathologist and her specialized treatment of tongue thrust as the creator and author of the "Stone Tongue Thrust Protocol: A Protocol for the Assessment and Treatment of Tongue Thrust". She gets satisfaction out of telling her childhood teachers that she found a way to make her "talking too much in class" pay off! Now she not only gets paid for talking but also for teaching others to do the same.

Through her transformation journey with Autoimmune Diseases, CallyRae found another passion through inspiring healthy living. Inspiring hope where there is hopelessness, confidence where there is fear, and joy where there is sadness has led her to transformation coaching with a lifestyle focus.

Whether as a Speech Language Pathologist or a Transformation Coach, CallyRae is innovative and eclectic. She loves to encourage and educate people about their potential and give them the tools to strive for more. She seems to gravitate to the challenges and seek for the solution. Whether it is a patient with a brain injury trying to rebuild their cognition; a student struggling to learn how to teach a complex client a new skill; or an individual who has given up because of their frustration with life: CallyRae will find a solution and offer hope.

You can follow CallyRae on social media for inspiration and ideas through her coaching page https://www.facebook.com/CallyRae2 or callystone1 on Instagram.

Printed in the United States
By Bookmasters